COLON HEALTH

Louise Tenney, M.H.

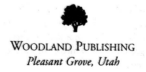

WOODLAND PUBLISHING
Pleasant Grove, Utah

CONTENTS

CONTENTS

COLON HEALTH

INTRODUCTION

As silly as it may sound, a healthy colon is the basis of a healthy body. In fact, most of us don't realize exactly how important a healthy colon is in maintaining optimal wellness.

Medical doctors used to focus on the health of the colon, but have actually regressed in recent years because of civilization's rush to abandon obsolete, outdated medical practices in favor of the latest and greatest pharmaceutical remedy or diagnostic gadget. Modern medical doctors just aren't as good as they used to be in assessing what really causes disease: an unhealthy colon. Colon health should be a primary concern in the quest for a healthy body.

A healthy body naturally depends on the maintenance of a healthy digestive system. Food is the primary source of fuel for the body and if the wrong foods are eaten, the body will not function properly. Nutrients, vitamins, minerals, enzymes, amino acids, carbohydrates and lipids found in the foods we eat provide the energy and resources that quite literally keep us alive.

Unfortunately, the foods we eat are also addled with toxins and unnecessary substances that hinder our body's ability to remove waster properly. In addition, every drip of water, every gulp of air, and every morsel of food we eat contains some toxic materials.

The body has natural means of dealing with the build-up of toxic materials in the body. Acute diseases—colds, flues, etc.—are actually a cleansing process in the body. If the symptoms of acute diseases are suppressed with medications or other means, the toxins may not entirely be removed (which may be the precursor to a more serious condition in the future.) Chronic conditions that develop may actually be a result of forbidding the body from ridding itself of toxic substances through acute disease.

In addition to acute disease, the body has another—and ultimately more important—method of "taking the trash out." A healthy colon is the foundation of a healthy body and learning natural methods to achieve colon health can be of utmost importance. Nutritious eating habits, cleansing diets, fiber sources, herbal remedies and nutritional supplements can all contribute to total well-being. Above all, we must all understand that a healthy body absolutely requires a healthy colon.

DIGESTION AND ASSIMILATION

Ultimately, the food we eat determines exactly how efficiently our entire body system works. Digestion is the body's first line of defense against foreign invaders that cause disease; in addition, the digestive system is also integral in supplying cells with much-needed nutrients and compounds.

Digestion, quite literally, is the breakdown of food at different locations in the body-the mouth, the stomach, the small and large intestine and the colon. Digestion involves assimilation of nutrients (and toxins) by blood and lymph vessels, where they are transported to every body cell for healing and rebuilding.

Along with nutrients, however, the blood and lymph vessels transport toxins to cells where they are allowed to accumulate and cause cell degeneration and oxidation. As a result, the immune system is significantly weakened and resistance to disease vanishes. The body becomes sluggish and heavier, the skin becomes blotchy and emotions unstable.

Causes of Digestive Problems

There are many factors that contribute to digestive disorders. These include overeating cooked food and not enough raw foods, constipation, wrong combination of food, caffeine, alcohol, tobacco, sugar and sweets, white flour product, stress, any imbalance in the body, lack of hydrochloric acid and enzymes, Candida overgrowth, colon and liver congestion, allergies, hiatal hernia, gallbladder problems, ulcers, heart problems

A Russian scientist named Kouchafoff found that after cooked food is eaten, white blood cells dramatically increased in the intestines. (Keep in mind that white blood cells are part of the immune system and always increase in number when there is a need to eliminate hostile invaders.) Apparently, a diet comprised primarily of cooked food can initiate the beginnings of inflammation or disease. Cooked food places an added burden on the immune system and also contributes to digestive disturbances.

The same Kouchafoff study found that eating raw food did not increase white cell response. Even more remarkable, a Swiss nutritionist discovered that eating raw vegetables before cooked food prevented the increase of white cells (Clark, 56). For example, a salad with endive or watercress included is very beneficial for digestion and will heal and repair the stomach.

Americans typically do themselves the most harm by the types and the amounts of food they eat. In order to break down food, the body uses acid in the stomach that is powerful enough to dissolve metal. This hydrochloric acid is used in the stomach to neutralize the inappropriate substances and toxins that enters our bodies through the food we eat every day. And on occasion, the stomach and its acid-based lines of defense breakdown and digestive malfunction occurs.

Nutrients for Proper Digestion

❑ *Digestive Enzymes* are essential in the digestion of any food. Acidophilus is important for proper bowel function. It helps to balance the normal flora of the intestinal tract.

❑ *Hydrochloric Acid* is necessary for the assimilation of vitamins and minerals; especially vitamin C and calcium.

❑ *B-Complex Vitamins* help promote a healthy digestive tract. They assist enzymes in the metabolism of proteins, fats and carbohydrates.

❑ *Sodium* is stored in the stomach wall and also in the joints. Sodium neutralizes acidity in the body. Sodium is needed when there is a deficiency of hydrochloric acid.

❑ *Calcium* is an essential mineral and if the stomach is low in hydrochloric acid, it will lead to decreased absorption of calcium and other vital minerals.

❑ *Fiber* is essential for proper digestion and elimination of food. It reduces the absorption of fat, inhibits bad estrogens from absorbing into the bloodstream, and helps maintain a healthy digestive tract.

Herbal Aids for Proper Digestion

❑ Capsicum, garlic, gentian, ginger, goldenseal, licorice, papaya juice or tablets, psyllium powder

❑ A lower bowel formula can stimulate daily bowel elimination as well as clean the built-up crust on the colon walls.

❑ Avoid over the counter synthetic antacids. There are natural remedies readily available in the form of herbs, digestive enzymes, acidophilus, and activated charcoal.

ENZYMES, AMINO ACIDS & ACIDOPHILUS

Enzymes are essential for life; without them, our body's ability to ward off disease is limited. These "spark plugs" of the human body are involved in nearly every biochemical function in the human body. They digest food, destroy parasites (worms, bacteria, etc.) and toxins that invade the body, and assist in the destruction of damaging free radicals before they wreak havoc on cellular structures. Simply put, without enzymes, the body would fall apart. The reason autoimmune diseases are so prevalent in modern times is because of the lack of enzymes in the human body. We simply are not getting enough of them anymore.

Amino Acids

In the past, amino acids have been very much ignored or neglected during intensive nutritional research. But today, amino acids are being recognized for their astonishing capabilities in restoring and maintaining good health. In fact, amino acid therapy has proven useful in ailments as wide-ranging as arthritis, anxiety, cancer, chronic fatigue, Candida, behavioral disorders, attention deficit disorder, anxiety, autoimmune diseases, chemical sensitivity, learning disorders, eating disorders, hypoglycemia, diabetes, cardiovascular diseases, seizures, headaches and chronic pain.

Most of the 23 identifiable amino acids can be manufactured by the body, but there are eight amino acids that must be supplied in the diet. They are isolecine, leucine, lysine, methionine, phenylalanine, threonine, tryptophan, and valine. And two amino acids, cysteine and tyrosine, which should also be classified also as "essential" because they are actual derivatives of the essential amino acids, methionine and phenylalanine.

In addition, there are two "nonessential" amino acids, histidine and arginine, that should be considered "essential" for young children. The body cannot meet the demands of histidine and arginine in children undergoing rapid growth.

Acidophilus

Each body has an ecosystem of sorts, with trillions of microorganisms making their home there. Acidophilus is one of these microorganisms and is actually a beneficial bacteria that flourish and live on the walls of the intestines and vagina. Acidophilus is necessary for proper digestion, assimilation and acts as a first line of defense in protecting the intestinal and vaginal tracts from infection and disease. Amazingly, acidophilus has the ability to change and adapt to any myriad of environmental changes inside the intestines.

Acidophilus helps to protect the body from an invasion of Candida and other germs that invade and live in the body. Lactobacillus acidophilus actually adheres to the walls of the instestines and the vagina and prevents disease-causing bacteria from taking hold. When the good acidophilus bacteria are compromised, there is suddenly room at the inn for the invading bacteria and they quickly take root.

Acidophilus also consumes all the food reserves available to microorganisms; when invading bacteria encounter regions were acidophilus are plentiful, the bad bacteria simply passes through without taking up residence. Acidophilus is also responsible for producing acetic acids which lower the natural pH in the intestines which discourages the growth of the other bacteria which flourish in a more acidic environment.

The intestinal and vaginal flora can be affected by various elements. The overuse of antibiotics, oral contraceptives, excessive sugar consumption, aspirin, antihistamines, cortisone, prednisone, coffee and stress all contribute to an imbalance in the bacterial flora of the gastrointestinal tract. When the friendly bacteria are outnumbered, detrimental substances may not be excreted from the body, which leads to unhealthy conditions.

Every day, we encounter and consume "bad" bacteria. When acidophilus is plentiful in the body, however, microorganism that invade the body with detrimental agendas are neutralized—defanged, if you will.

CONSTIPATION

Constipation is a very serious health threat with far-reaching consequences. It is a common, but very dangerous, ailment that afflicts every segment of our society. Bowel dysfunction can manifest itself in many ways, but the bottom line (no pun intended) is that a clean and efficiently functioning colon is absolutely essential to our health, well-being and longevity.

The current technical definition of constipation makes reference to a decrease in bowel movements or difficulty in the formation or passage of the stool. While this definition may be technically correct it is incomplete and fails to explain all of the ramifications of a dysfunctional colon. In reality, several kinds of constipation exist and most of us unknowingly suffer from one form of this malady or another. John Harvey Kellogg, M.D. in his book *Colon Hygiene* describes three forms of constipation:

SIMPLE CONSTIPATION: This condition arises when the elimination of the bowel content is not complete. Consequently, fecal matter remains in the bowels and gradually builds up and adheres to the colon wall. This condition can be the consequence of irregular eating schedules, overeating cooked food, lack of exercise and neglecting the urge to eliminate. This condition may signal the beginning of chronic constipation and may be a significant precursor to many of the ailments that plague mankind.

CUMULATIVE CONSTIPATION: This is considered the most common form of constipation. It is mostly confined to the lower part of the colon and is due to lazy peristaltic action. The purpose of peristaltic waves—the urge to pass a bowel movement—is to propel the contents of the colon from the cecum to the rectum for eventual elimination. Lack of normal bowel action can cause injury to the colon walls and the ileocecal valve in the large intestine. As a result of cumulative constipation, straining is usually necessary to eliminate fecal matter from the body. This straining can eventually cause hemorrhoids (internal and external), varicose veins, lower back pain and many other symptoms.

LATENT CONSTIPATION: This type of constipation typically occurs in people who suffer from chronic disease. Latent constipation takes years to develop and most people are not aware of its presence because the bowels move regularly. Symptoms of this kind of constipation are numerous and include fatigue, headaches, bad breath, appendicitis, colitis, PMS, anxiety, and depression—and that is just the beginning of the list. (Kellogg, 195-200).

DIARRHEA: It may seem strange that diarrhea is listed as a type of constipation, but the malady is caused by an irritation in the colon. Chronic diarrhea can occur when certain irritants adhere to the bowel walls and cannot be eliminated. The bowel reacts negatively and forces waste out as quickly as possible, resulting in diarrhea. Hardened bowel residue can be loosened and removed with herbal formulas.

Causes of Constipation

There can be many causes of constipation. These include a lack of dietary fiber; slow transit time; bowel adhesions due to infected or deranged mucus membranes of the bowel wall; stretched colon from food overload; ileocecal valve incontinence; lack of exercise; drinking too little water; poor posture; hemorrhoids; weak bowel muscles; nervous disorders; a lack of hydrochloric acid and digestive enzymes

In addition to the above causes, constipation can be caused by pregnancy, neurological and endocrine disorders, diabetes, an underactive thyroid gland and some medications. Some of these constipation-causing drugs include codeine (or other high-potency pain killers), antacids with aluminum, iron tablets, and some narcotics and antidepressants. Stress and anxiety have also been linked to constipation. A physical obstruction in the bowel caused by a stricture, tumor or diverticulosis may result in constipation as well. An enlarged prostate gland or the presence of endometriosis may put pressure on the rectum, subsequently decreasing bowel activity.

Symptoms of Constipation

Painful bowel movements due to the hardness of the stool; the inability to have a complete bowel movement; bloating and gas; a tender or distended abdomen; a feeling of sluggishness; the development of hemorrhoids; indigestion; insomnia; depression or anxiety.

Preventing Constipation.

Adding fiber to the diet in combination with plenty of raw fruits and vegetables can work fabulously to prevent constipation. The amount of fiber recommended for anyone who suffers from constipation is 40 grams per day, which can be easily found in cereal sources of fiber combined with fruits and vegetables. Remember, however, that it is important to increase your water intake anytime your fiber consumption goes up.

LEAKY GUT SYNDROME

Dr. Sherry A. Rogers, M.D., explains leaky gut syndrome: "The leaky gut syndrome is a poorly recognized, but extremely common problem that is seldom tested for. It represents a hyperpermeable intestinal lining. In other words, large spaces develop between the cells of the gut wall and bacteria, toxins and food leak in." (*Let's Live*, April 1995, 34-35)

If the lining of the intestinal tract becomes more permeable than normal, it can lead to serious health concerns. The large spaces that develop between the cells of the gut wall allow toxic material to enter the bloodstream. Under normal conditions these toxic substances will be eliminated, but when leaky gut syndrome occurs, parasites, bacteria, fungi, toxins, fats and other foreign matter not normally absorbed enter the bloodstream. These microbes can put a strain on the liver's ability to detoxify.

When antibodies are released due to leaky gut syndrome, they can attach to various body tissues leading to an inflammatory response. If the inflammation occurs in a joint, rheumatoid arthritis may result. If the antibodies attack the gut lining, various gastrointestinal problems can develop such as Crohn's disease or colitis. Other associated problems include migraines, eczema, and immune problems. The body's furious antibody response can produce leaky gut-like symptoms in just about any organ or area of the body.

Causes of Leaky Gut Syndrome

Leaky gut syndrome can be caused by a number of factors basically associated with today's lifestyle. The major problem occurs with an inflammation of the gut lining leading to hypermeability. This may result because of the following:

Antibiotics, poor diet, alcohol and caffeine, NSAIDS (nonsteroidal anti-inflammatory drugs), enzyme deficiencies, chemicals, parasite infection, molds and fungus consumption from grains and fruits, symptoms, fatigue, low-grade fever, frequent colds, flu, infections, aches and pains, fungal disease, nausea after eating, food intolerances and allergies, chemical sensitivities, abdominal pain, abdominal distention, diarrhea, skin rashes, toxic feelings, cognitive and memory deficits, shortness of breath, difficulty exercising

Diseases associated with Leaky Gut Syndrome

Inflammatory bowel syndrome, acne, eczema, psoriasis, AIDS, cystic fibrosis, liver disease, rheumatoid arthritis, asthma, celiac disease, lupus, fibromyalgia, chronic fatigue syndrome, autism, food and chemical sensitivities

Dietary Guidelines

❏ The following vegetable juice combinations will assist in ridding the body of leaky gut syndrome:
  • Carrot, celery, and endive

- Carrot, parsley, and cabbage,
- Ginger, parsley, garlic, carrots and celery
Fasting on these juices two to three days a week will help to speed the healing process of the digestive tract.
❑ Thermos cooked grains are healing on the digestive tract. They are rich in enzymes, vitamins, minerals and protein. This slow-cooking process prevents destruction of the vital enzymes.
❑ Drink plenty of liquids including pure water, electrolyte drinks without added sugar, fruit juices diluted with pure water, and almond milk which is rich in calcium, magnesium and protein. Almond milk can be used be added to fruit drinks.
❑ Millet, buckwheat and basmati brown rice can be eaten for breakfast. They are easy for the body to digest and very nourishing.
❑ Raw vegetables and fruits, steams vegetables, yams and avocados are all helpful in healing the digestive tract.

Nutritional Supplements

Acidophilus, plant digestive enzymes, vitamin A (beta-carotene), B-complex, vitamin C with bioflavonoids, antioxidants, calcium/magnesium, essential fatty acids (flax seed oil, salmon oil, evening primrose oil, blue-green algae

Herbal Aids

Aloe vera juice, cat's claw, grapeseed extract, pau d'arco, licorice, goldenseal, slippery elm, comfrey

PARASITES AND WORMS

Parasites and worms are scavengers and organisms that live within, upon or at the expense of another organism (known as the host) without contributing to the survival of the host. They can reside in the gastrointestinal tract and feed on toxins and waste material in the body. The most common types include round-worms (hookworms, pinworms and threadworms) and tape-worms. The main problem is that the parasites expel waste material into the host that can be extremely toxic and even deadly.

The infestation of parasites are causing many diseases that have baffled doctors. Improper sanitation measures have resulted in people ingesting contaminated food, water and dirt. If the body is free of toxins with adequate amounts of hydrochloric acid being produced, it can destroy parasites and worms and their larva. However, a diet rich in fat, starch and sugar (sound familiar?) provides food for parasites and worms.

Parasites and worms may be associated with many diseases. But unfortunately most medical professionals never even check for them. They may be associated with colon disorders, AIDS, some types of cancer, chronic fatigue syndrome, and Candida.

Worms and parasites can be contracted in many different ways. An individual may unknowingly come in contact with waste material that is contaminated. Walking barefoot on contaminated soil can lead to infestation. Ingestion of larvae or eggs from handling meat or partially cooked meat may be the cause.

Another parasite, *Giardia lamblia*, a microscopic organism has been found in some municipal drinking water. It is often found in streams and lakes and then introduced into the drinking water supplies. It is generally left behind by animal waste.

Frequent use of antibiotics, a poor diet, other medications, and even stress can reduce beneficial intestinal flora and provide an environment for parasites and worms to thrive.

Symptoms of Parasitic Infection

Poor absorption of nutrients, abdominal pain, loss of appetite, weight loss, diarrhea, anemia, colon disorders such as ileocecal valve syndrome, rectal itching, growth problems in children, diminished immune function, constipation, gas and bloating, fatigue, colitis, headaches

Dietary Guidelines

❏ Eat a high fiber diet full of raw vegetables, fruits and whole grains.

❏ Pumpkin seeds, pomegranate seeds, sesame seeds and figs can help rid the body of parasites and worms.

❏ Garlic, onions, cabbage and carrots contain sulfur which aids in expelling parasites from the body.

❏ Avoid sugar, refined foods, white flour products, chocolate, alcohol, tobacco and caffeine.

❏ Limit or avoid entirely meat products, especially pork. If meat is eaten, make sure it is fully cooked.

❏ Hydrochloric Acid and digestive enzymes are very important. The hydrochloric acid helps to kill the parasites when sufficient supplies are available.

❏ Blood, colon and liver cleansers are necessary to get rid of the toxins that feed parasites and worms.

Nutritional Supplements

Multivitamin/mineral supplement, B-complex vitamins, vitamin C with bioflavonoids, zinc, acidophilus, essential fatty acids

Herbal Aids

Garlic, black walnut, burdock, echinacea, goldenseal, aloe vera juice, grapeseed extract, pumpkin seed

HIATAL HERNIA

The "hiatus" in the body is a hole in the diaphragm where the esophagus passes to join the top of the stomach. A "hiatal" hernia occurs when the stomach inches its way into that hole and protrudes into the diaphragm (of course, "hernia" refers to a weakened area of the body or stretched muscle.)

With a herniated muscle (diaphragm), the stomach is allowed to creep upward through the diaphragm. Small hernias may go undetected but may cause various symptoms include heartburn and belching. This is a common problem among the elderly, and it is estimated that up to 50 percent of the population over the age of 40 suffer from a lessened version this condition.

Symptoms of Hiatal Hernia

Symptoms of hiatal hernia center around chronic heartburn and belching. Stomach acid sometimes comes up into the throat, causing a burning and a discomfort in the chest and throat. Other symptoms of hiatal hernia could include belching, heartburn, bloating, intestinal gas, regurgitation, nausea, vomiting, diarrhea, constipation, fatigue, allergies, burning in upper chest, pressure below breastbone, dizziness, anxiety

Dietary Guidelines

❑ Drink large glasses of water throughout the day.
❑ Eat several small meals a day in a calm environment and never eat within two hours of bedtime..
❑ Add more grains to the diet.
❑ Eat more fruit, vegetables and natural foods and less meat.
❑ Avoid fat and fried foods.
❑ Avoid coffee, tea, alcohol, cola and smoking.

Nutritional Supplements

Antioxidants, zinc, vitamin A, B-complex vitamins, vitamin C, minerals, chlorophyll, coenzyme Q10, papaya enzyme

Herbal Aids

Aloe vera, gentian, ginger, goldenseal, slippery elm, marshmallow root

ILEOCECAL VALVE SYNDROME

The ileocecal valve is made up of sphincter muscles that close the ileum (the point where the small intestine empties into the ascending colon—or "jejunum"). Basically, the ileocecal valve prevents toxins and other materials that are released by the appendix—which is close to the opening into the small intestine—from entering into the small intestine.

In addition, the ileocecal valve helps to keep the digested material in the small intestine until the all the nutrients have been absorbed. When the food residue is ready for elimination, the small intestine mixes it with mucus, bile and other excretions and releases it systematically through the ileocecal vale into the large intestine. This prevents an overload of material for the body to eliminate.

Ileocecal valve syndrome occurs when the toxic material of the colon is permitted to enter back into the small intestine, where it is rapidly reabsorbed, leading to infection and disease.

Symptoms of Ileocecal Valve Syndrome

Constipation, diarrhea, fatigue, irregular bowel movements, lower right bowel tenderness, acne, immune weakness, migraines, duodenal ulcers

Dietary Guidelines

❑ Eat a diet high in fiber including whole grains. Soak the grains and cook to avoid irritating the valve.

❑ Avoid foods that cause constipation like dairy products, meat, bananas, etc.

❑ Eat stewed prunes, figs and raisins for breakfast.

❑ Add more fresh fruits and vegetables to the diet. The softer raw vegetables such as leaf lettuce, spinach, avocados, sprouts and tomatoes should be used at first.

❑ Reduce the amount of meat eaten.

❏ Take a fiber supplement to avoid constipation.

❏ Fasting on these juices two to three days a week will help to speed the healing process of the digestive tract.

❏ Thermos-cooked grains are healing on the digestive tract. They are rich in enzymes, vitamins, minerals and protein. This slow cooking process prevents destruction of the vital enzymes.

❏ Millet, buckwheat and basmati brown rice can be eaten for breakfast. They are easy for the body to digest and very nourishing.

❏ Raw vegetables and fruits, steamed vegetables, yams and avocados are all helpful in healing the digestive tract.

Nutritional Supplements

Antioxidants, vitamin A (beta-carotene), B-complex, vitamin C with bioflavonoids, calcium/magnesium, essential fatty acids, blue-green algae, acidophilus, plant digestive enzymes

Herbal Aids

Aloe vera juice, cat's claw, grapeseed extract, pau d'arco, licorice, goldenseal, slippery elm, comfrey

ALLERGIES

Allergies are the result of an immune system that is categorically weakened by a poor diet, polluted air, chemicals and other toxic substances. In addition, there are usually several reasons allergies develop. As a result, physicians have difficulty properly identifying what is causing the allergy and they end up only treating one allergy with drug therapy that masks the true problem.

Amazingly, the colon can contribute in the fight against allergies. Eating a lot of junk food, sugar, meat, and nutritionally poor food along with the toxins in the environment can cause the colon to become congested or constipated. When this constipation occurs, damaging chemicals and toxins reenter the bloodstream and force the immune system into action. Allergic substances, which are not as dangerous as the toxins and poisons we eat, are ignored by an immune system that is fighting off invasive compounds elsewhere in the body.

Symptoms of Allergies

Hives, rashes, inflammation, watery eyes, itching, nasal congestion, sneezing, runny nose, sinusitis, diarrhea, constipation, arthritis, headache, irritability, lethargy, hyperactivity, excessive gas, colitis, canker sores, belching, heartburn, indigestion, eczema

Dietary Guidelines to Prevent Allergies

❏ A cleansing diet can help to eliminate toxins from the blood.

❏ Digestive enzymes and hydrochloric acid can help with the digestion and absorption of food.

❏ Juice fasting with carrot, celery and raw apple juice may be beneficial.

❏ Colon cleansing using gentle herbs can help with constipation.

❏ Make sure the liver is healthy by using a liver cleanse. The liver is responsible for ridding the body of accumulated toxins. It also helps to produce histamines which protects the body against allergies.

❏ Avoid foods with additives. Stay away from FD&C yellow no. 5 dyes, along with BHT-BHA, benzoates, annatto, eucayptol, monosodium glutamate and vanillin.

❏ Eliminate foods that cause allergies such as wheat, eggs, dairy products, caffeine, chocolate, shellfish, strawberries, tomatoes and citrus fruits. After approximately four weeks, the foods can be reintroduced one at a time. Stay away from foods that offer no nutritional value.

Nutritional Supplements

Muiti-mineral vitamin supplement, vitamin C with bioflavonoids, vitamin A and beta-carotene, calcium with magnesium, potassium, B-complex vitamins, digestive enzyme combination, quercentin, tyrosine, acidophilus, coenzyme Q10 and germanium

Herbal Aids

Bee pollen, blessed thistle, pleurisy root, burdock, garlic, echinacea, kelp, ephedra, goldenseal root, marshmallow, lobelia

AUTOINTOXICATION

The health of the colon is essential for a healthy body. Many medical doctors in the past—as well as some health-oriented doctors today—know that the health of the colon can determine the health of the body, mind and nervous system. Autointoxication; toxemia, and constipation can lead to nervous disorders. Constipation may even be an underlying cause of some cases of depression, mood swings, despair, stress, anxiety, insomnia or even strokes.

In June, 1917, an article, titled entitled "Symptomatology of the Nervous System In Chronic Intestinal Toxemia," was read at the 68th annual session of the American Medical Association in New York City. It was written by G. Reese Satterlee, M.D. and Watson W. Eldridge, M.D., and reported that 518 cases of mental symptoms ranging from mental sluggishness to hallucinations were relieved through eliminating intestinal toxemia (Satterlee, 1414).

During periods of emotional distress the stomach becomes irritated and the stomach tightens up. Consequently, the blood supply is unable to reach the stomach lining and congestion and inflammation results. If this is allowed to continue, the cells of the stomach lining eventually die from lack of nourishment, setting the stage for a grim lineup of ailments: ulcers, colitis, appendicitis—and even cancer.

Constipation, which leads to a toxic colon, can overburden the liver. The liver is unable to filter out the increased amounts of toxins effectively, resulting in brain and nervous system disorders.

Dietary Guidelines

❏ Eat foods that offer nutritional support to the body.
❏ Add more vegetables, fruits and whole grains to the diet.
❏ Avoid foods that cause stress on the body such as alcohol, tobacco, caffeine, sugar products and refined foods.

Nutritional Supplements

Vitamin/mineral supplement with antioxidants, B-complex vitamins with extra B12 and B6, vitamin C with bioflavonoids, calcium/magnesium

Herbal Aids

Black cohosh, lady's slipper, skullcap, gotu kola, kava kava, burdock, oatstraw, passionflower, prickly ash, ginger, ginkgo, bee pollen, ginseng, licorice, wood betony

CANDIDA

Candida is a normally occurring fungus that lives in the mucous membranes, especially in the digestive tract and vagina. It can also be found in the sinuses, ear canals, and genito-urinary tract. The body can handle normal amounts of this fungus, but in large amounts, it is detrimental to digestive health. Under normal conditions the yeasts live in harmony with other organisms in the intestinal flora. Candidiasis (overgrowth of *Candida albicans*) is a more common condition in women of childbearing years though it can even infect infants and children.

Problems arise when the body's natural immune function is compromised because of various conditions like a lack of sleep, poor diet, stress, drugs, antibiotics, birth control pills, lack of exercise and environmental pollutants. Anything that weakens the immune system will in turn encourage the growth of Candida. A strong and healthy immune system will still contain Candida in relatively small amounts. Only when the immune system falters does Candida increase in the body.

Symptoms of Candida

Fatigue, sore throat, bad breath, chronic infections, thyroid problems, panic attacks, migraine headaches, swollen glands, digestive disorders, constipation, depression, indigestion, feeling spaced-out

Dietary Guidelines

❏ Eliminate sugar, honey, white flour products, yeast breads, wine, beer, fruit juices, cheese, mushrooms, junk food, refined foods, vinegar products and limit fruit to small amounts until the yeast is under control.
❏ Millet, brown rice and whole grains and vegetables are good.
❏ Beans are a good source of protein.
❏ Almonds and nuts are good, but avoid peanuts.
❏ A great drink can be made from carrots, parsley, garlic and ginger.
❏ Add fiber to the diet—it helps to cleanse the colon and eliminate toxins.

Nutritional Supplements

Vitamin A and beta-carotene, vitamin C with bioflavonoids, B-complex vitamins, vitamin E, multi-vitamin and mineral supplement, acidophilus, blue-green algae, caprylic acid, olive oil, digestive enzymes, coenzyme Q10

Herbal Aids

Cat's claw, pau d'arco, garlic, barberry, echinacea, dong quai

CLEANSING FOR A HEALTHY BODY

In order to make health a way of life, eating patterns need to be changed. Restoring health to the body is impossible without cleansing the colon, blood and lymphatic systems. Poor eating habits are the main reason the body is laden with toxins and poisons. The body can heal itself, but a cleansing and eliminating program is necessary to retain health and in allowing the body to heal.

Suggested Transition Diet

Before breakfast you can use supplements that are needed for whatever condition you have. If you have Candida, for exmaple, take acidophilus first thing in the morning on an empty stomach, and use appropriate nutrients, foods and herbs that go along with Candida. If you have hypoglycemia, eat the appropriate diet, supplements, herbs to strengthen the body to overcome this condition.

Breakfast should consist of fruits such as cantaloupe, watermelon, peaches, grapes, pears, apricots, apples or citrus fruit. After an hour use a protein drink, thermos cereal, millet or a brown rice dish. Fresh fruit juices or vegetable juices can also be use; they should always be diluted with half pure water.

Lunch can consist of salads using sprouts of all kinds, grain soups, steamed and raw vegetables. Use brown rice and millet dishes. You can also drink fresh tomato vegetable cocktail juices.

Dinner should be lighter than breakfast and lunch. You can drink fresh vegetable juices, steamed vegetables, baked potatoes, brown rice and millet dishes along with fresh salads.

Cleansing Diet (from the Seneca indians)

The reason this diet is beneficial is the first day the colon is cleansed. The second day toxins are released. Salt and excessive calcium deposits in the muscles, tissues and organs are eliminated. The third day the digestive tract is supplied with healthy, mineral rich bulk. The fourth day the blood, lymph and organs are cleansed.

FIRST DAY: Eat fruit, all you want, such as apples, berries, watermelon, pears, cherries, apricots but no bananas.

SECOND DAY: Drink all the herb teas you want such as chamomile, raspberry, spearmint, hyssop, Pau d'Arco, and red clover blends. If you sweeten the tea, use pure maple syrup.

THIRD DAY: Eat all the vegetables you want; eat them raw, steamed or both.

FOURTH DAY: Make a pan of vegetable broth using cauliflower, cabbage, onion, green pepper, parsley or whatever you have on hand. Season with natural salt or vegetable seasoning. Drink only the rich mineral broth all day.

Cleansing the Liver

❑ Take a hydrochloric acid formula before meals.

❑ Take plant digestive enzymes during or after the meal.

❑ Goats whey powder is rich in minerals, especially natural sodium, which will help heal and repair the digestive tract. Use a tablespoon three times a day.

❑ Take a combination with digestive herbs. Herbal formulas will supply nutrients to help stimulate and increase enzyme activity.

❑ Use an herbal lower bowel formula to help cleanse the colon.

❑ Take an herbal supplement to help strengthen and repair the liver.

❑ Main herbs include gentian, licorice, goldenseal, fennel, blue green algae, barley grass, catnip and alfalfa

❑ Assisting herbs include Oregon grape, milk thistle, dandelion, barberry, cruciferous vegetables, cardamon, and barberry

❑ Transporting herbs include capsicum, ginger, turmeric, lobelia, aloe vera, papaya, and peppermint

Cleansing the Kidneys

❑ Minerals will help restore health to the kidneys.

❑ A potassium formula and goats whey powder will heal the entire digestive tract as well as the kidneys.

❑ Take an herbal kidney cleansing and strengthening formula.

❑ Main herbs include oatstraw, cornsilk, uva ursi, goldenseal, Pau d'Arco, dandelion, horsetail, juniper, cranberry powder, and watermelon seeds *Assisting herbs include: marshmallow, kelp, comfrey, echinacea, mullein, and slippery elm.

❑ Transporting herbs include lobelia, ginger, peppermint, prickly ash, and capsicum

❑ Acidophilus helps prevent infections and increases friendly bacteria.

❑ Chlorophyll and blue-green algae clean and heal infections and blood.

Cleansing the Colon

❑ Proper digestion will help speed the colon cleanse.

❑ An herbal cleansing tea is one way to get started on a colon cleanse.

❑ An herbal fiber formula is essential.

❑ A lower bowel cleanser is very important to help clean and loosen encrusted material on the colon walls.

❑ Main herbs are cascara sagrada, butternut bark, rhubarb, and burdock.

❑ Assisting herbs include fenugreek, slipper elm, licorice, kelp, Irish moss, blue green algae or other chlorophyll sources, or goldenseal.

❑ Transporting herbs are lobelia, capsicum, fennel, ginger and peppermint.

❑ The following herbs should used to rebuild and strengthen the colon walls bee pollen, kelp, blue green algae, slippery elm, comfrey, marshmallow, aloe vera juice and papaya.

Cleansing the Lungs

❑ Follow guidelines for digestion, liver and colon cleansing.
❑ Take a formula for cleansing and strengthening the lungs.
❑ Main herbs include ephedra, fenugreek, mullein, marshmallow, boneset, echinacea, chlorophyll or use other green sources, and elecampane
❑ Assisting herbs are: myrrh, licorice, pleurisy, hops, skullcap, comfrey, plantain, and eucalyptus.
❑ Transporting herbs are lobelia, capsicum, ginger, and prickly ash.

Cleansing the Skin

❑ Colon, liver, kidney and blood cleansers are needed when cleansing the skin.
❑ Skin brushing will help speed the cleansing of the skin. Use natural cleansers for the skin to prevent clogging up the pores and preventing skin elimination.
❑ Faulty fat metabolism is a cause of most skin diseases. Foods rich in omega-3 and gamma-linoleic acids will help remedy this problem.
❑ Herbal formulas for the cleansing the skin can help.
❑ Main herbs are red clover, yellow dock, sarsparilla, burdock, yarrow, alfalfa, kelp, marshmallow, and sassafras
❑ Assisting herbs include chlorophyll sources, rose hips, fenugreek, licorice, and thyme.
❑ Transporting herbs are ginger, cloves, fennel, lobelia, cayenne, and rosemary.

Cleansing the Blood and Lymphatics

❑ Eat healthy foods.

❑ Hydrochloric acid and digestive enzymes improve and repair the digestive system.

❑ Occasional fasting is necessary to help the body heal itself.

❑ Use an herbal formula to help cleanse the blood.

❑ Main herbs are red clover, Pau d'Arco, chaparral, echinacea, burdock, Oregon grape, goldenseal, ho shou wu, milk thistle, and suma.

❑ Assisting herbs are sheep sorrel, peach bark, licorice, astragalus, hyssop, myrrh gum, sarsaparilla, dandelion, wild yam, yellow dock, and cat's claw.

❑ Transporting herbs include prickly ash, ginger, lobelia, capsicum, kelp, fennel, cinnamon, and peppermint.

Cleansing the Body of Parasites and Worms

❑ Hydrochloric acid and digestive enzymes are very important.

❑ Blood, colon and liver cleansers are necessary to get rid of the toxins that parasites and worms feed on.

❑ Eliminate white flour and sugar products. Eat a diet using fresh and steamed vegetables. Salads are important but need to be rinsed in apple cider vinegar to kill the larva.

❑ Take an herbal formula to destroy and expel worms from the body.

❑ Main herbs are black walnut hulls, wormwood, garlic, cloves, chaparral, gentian, pumpkin seeds, tea tree oil, cascara sagrada, aloe vera, and licorice

❑ Assisting herbs are rhubarb, barberry, gentian, blue green algae, thyme, calendula, and alfalfa

❑ Transporting herbs include lobelia, ginger, prickly ash, peppermint, and capsicum.

CONCLUSION

Nutritional supplements are increasing in popularity. As more individuals become aware of the their nutritional deficiencies, natural approaches to replenishing the body are being sought. The digestive system has often been overlooked as a factor in overall body health. If food and supplements are not absorbed and assimilated, the nutrients may not reach the bloodstream to nourish the entire body.

Colon health is more important than most people realize. The digestive process is directly related to the health of the body, immune system function and even longevity. When any disease occurs, it is basic to look to the colon first for treatment. Following the example of doctors from the past, may assist in promoting future health.

Start by understanding what it means to have a healthy colon. Gradually add fiber, nutritional supplements, and herbal helps along with a change in diet. Slowly change eating habits. It does not have to happen overnight. Eliminate unhealthy, nutrition robbing foods from the diet. Stress whole grain foods, fruits and vegetables.

We all need to take a look at our lifestyle habits and examine areas that need improvement. Most of us can certainly improve on the food we eat and feed our families. Small changes may mean significant improvement in health. Taking action now may mean a longer, healthier and happier life.

BIBLIOGRAPHY

Balch, James F., M.D. and Phyllis A. Balch, Prescription For Nutritional Healing (Garden City Park, N.Y.: Avery Publishing Group, 1997).

Bateson-Koch, Carolee, Allergies, Disease in Disguise (Burnaby, B.C. Canada: Alive Books, 1994).

Brown, Donald J. Herbal Prescription For Better Health (Rocklin, CA: Prima Publishing, 1996).

Castleman, Michael, Nature's Cures. (Emmaus, Pennsylvania: Rodale Press, Inc., 1996), 176.

Challem, Jack "Good Bacteria that Fight the Bad," Let's Live. October, 1995 55.

Chichoke, Anthony J., Enzymes and Enzyme Therapy (New Cannan, Connecticut: Keats Publishing, 1994).

Christopher, John R., Regenerative Diet (Springville, UT: Christopher Publications, 1982).

Clark, Linda, The New Way To Eat (Millbrae, CA: Celestial Arts, 1980)

Cohen, M.L. "Epidemiology of drug resistance: implications for a post-antimicrobial era," Science, (1992; 257) 1050-1055.

Elkins, Rita, The Complete Fiber Fact Book (Pleasant Grove, UT: Woodland Publishing, Inc., 1996).

Elkins, Rita, The Complete Home Health Advisor (Pleasant Grove, UT: Woodland Publishing, Inc., 1994).

Fitch, William E., M.D., "Putrefactive Intestinal Toxemia,"Medical Journal and Record (132) (August 20, 1930): 189.

Galland, Leo, M.D., Superimmunity for Kids (N.Y.: Copestone Press, Inc., 1988).

Gittleman, Ann Louise, Guess What Came To Dinner (Garden City Park, N.Y.: Avery Publishing, Inc., 1993).

Harrison, Lewis, The Complete Book of Fats and Oils (Garden City Park, N.Y.: Avery Publishing, 1990).

Hausman, Patricia and Judith Benn Hurley, The Healing Foods (Emmaus, Pennsylvania: Rodale Press, 1989)

Hawley, Clark W. M.D., "Autointoxication and Eye Diseases," Opthamology Magazine 10 (14) (1914): 663-74.

Hobbs, Christopher, Foundations of Health (Capitola, CA: Botanica Press, 1992).

Jensen, Bernard, Tissue Cleansing Through Bowel Management (Escondido, CA: Bernard Jensen Enterprises, 1993).

Keji, C. and S. Jun, "Progress of research of ischemic stroke treated with Chinese medicine," Journal of Traditional Chinese Medicine. (12) (1992): 204-10.

Kellogg, John Harvey, M.D., Colon Hygiene (Good Health Publishing Co., 1916).

Kritchevsky, David, Charles Bonfield and James W. Anderson, Eds., Dietary Fiber. (New York: Plenum Press, 1988, 140).

Lane, Sir. W. Arbuthnot, M.D.,The Prevention of the Diseases Peculiar to Civilization (N.Y.: Foundation for Alternative Cancer Therapies, revised 1981).

Lindlahr, Henry, M.D., Philosophy of Natural Therapeutics (Chicago: Lindlahr, 1918).

Livingston-Wheeler, Virginia, M.D., The Conquest of Cancer (N.Y.: Franklin Watts, 1984).

Michnovicz, Jon J., How To Reduce Your Risk of Breast Cancer (N.Y.: Warner Books, 1994)

Monte, Tom, World Medicine, The East West guide To Healing Your Body (N.Y.:

Putnam Publishing Group, 1993).

Murray, Michael T. Healing With Whole Foods (Rocklin, CA: Prima Publishing, 1993 22).

Page, Linda Rector, How to be Your Own Herbal Pharmacist (1991).

Pitchford, Paul, Healing With Whole foods (Berkeley, CA: North Atlantic Books, 1993).

Rogers, Sherry A., M.D., Let's Live, April 1995, 34-35.

Rogers, Sherry A., M.D., Wellness Against All Odds (Syracuse, NY: Prestige Publishing, 1994).

Rona, Zoltan P., M.D., Return To The Joy Of Health (Burnaby, B.C. Canada: Alive Books, 1995).

Satterlee, Reese M.D. and Watson W. Eldridge, M.D. "Symptomatology of the Nervous System In Chronic Intestinal Toxemia," Journal of the American Medical Association 69 (17) (1917): 1414.

Scheer, James F., "Acidophilus, Nautre's Antibiotic," Better Nutrition For Today's Living, August, 1993, 34.

Simone, Charles B., M.D., Cancer and Nutrition (Garden City Park, N.Y.: Avery Publishing, 1992).

Somer, Elizabeth, Nutrition For Women, The Complete Guide. (New York: Henry Holt and Company, 1993) 382-84..

Story, J.A., "Dietary fiber and lipid metabolism," Medical Aspects of Dietary Fiber, (New York: Plenum Medical, 1980, 138).

Stucky, J.M., M.D., "Intestinal Intoxication," Journal of the American Medicalk Association Oct. 9, 1909.

Synnott, Martin J., M.D. Intestinal Toxemia in Diagnosis and Treatment (N.Y.: A.R. Elliot Publishing Co., 1932).

Tenney, Louise, Encyclopedia of Natural Remedies (Pleasant Grove, UT: Woodland Publishing, Inc., 1995).

Tenney, Louise, The Natural Guide To Colon Health (Pleasant Grove, UT: Woodland Publishing, Inc. 1997).

Tenney, Louise, Today's Herbal Health For Women (Pleasant Grove, UT: Woodland Publishing, Inc., 1996).

Tenney, Louise, Today's Herbal Health (Pleasant Grove, UT: Woodland Publishing, Inc., 1997).

Tenney, Louise, Nutritional Guide (Pleasant Grove, UT: Woodland Publishing, Inc., 1994).

A. Vogel, M.D., "Improved Liver Function," Bestways, Sept. 1986, 31.

Willet, et al, "Reation of meat, fat and fiber intake to the risk of colon cancer in a prospective study among women." New England Journal of Medicine (323):1664-72.

Yiamouyiannis, John, M.D. Flouride and the Aging Factor (Delaware, Ohio: Health Action Press, 1993).